The Amazing Fish and Meat Mediterranean Cookbook

Delicious Recipes to Stay Fit and Enjoy Your Diet

Raymond Morton

Table of contents

4

Turkey and Savoy Cabbage

Prep time: 10 minutes I **Cooking time:** 35 minutes I
Servings: 4

Ingredients:

- 1 big turkey breast, skinless, boneless and cubed
- 1 cup chicken stock
- 1 tablespoon coconut oil, melted
- 1 Savoy cabbage, shredded
- 1 teaspoon chili powder
- 1 teaspoon sweet paprika
- 1 garlic clove, minced
- 1 yellow onion, chopped
- A pinch of salt and black pepper

Directions:

1. Heat up a pan with the oil over medium heat, add the meat and brown for 5 minutes.
2. Add the garlic and the onion, toss and sauté for 5 minutes more.
3. Add the cabbage and the other ingredients, toss, bring to a simmer and cook over medium heat for 25 minutes.
4. Divide everything between plates and serve.

Nutrition info per serving: calories 299, fat 14.5, fiber 5, carbs 8.8, protein 12.6

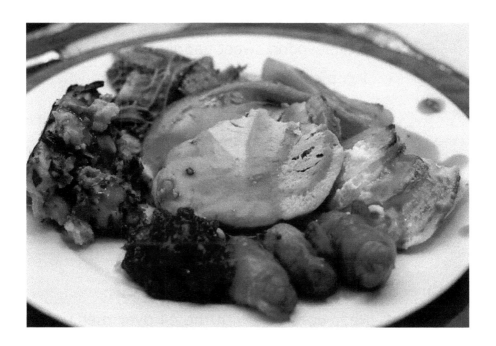

Chicken and Scallions

Prep time: 10 minutes I **Cooking time:** 30 minutes I
Servings: 4

Ingredients:

- 1 pound chicken breast, skinless, boneless and sliced
- 4 scallions, chopped
- 1 tablespoon olive oil
- 1 tablespoon sweet paprika
- 1 cup chicken stock
- 1 tablespoon ginger, grated
- 1 teaspoon oregano, dried
- 1 teaspoon cumin, ground
- 1 teaspoon allspice, ground
- ½ cup cilantro, chopped
- A pinch of black pepper

Directions:

1. Heat up a pan with the oil over medium heat, add the scallions and the meat and brown for 5 minutes.
2. Add the rest of the ingredients, toss, introduce in the oven and bake at 390 degrees F for 25 minutes.

3. Divide the chicken and scallions mix between plates and serve.

Nutrition info per serving: calories 295, fat 12.5, fiber 6.9, carbs 22.4, protein 15.6

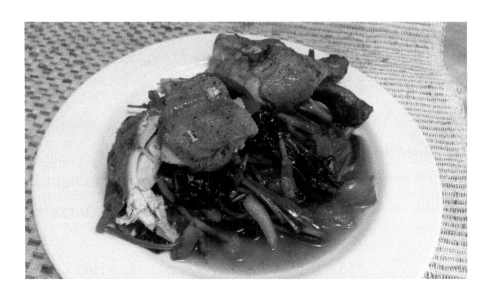

Chicken and Basil Mustard Sauce

Prep time: 10 minutes I **Cooking time:** 35 minutes I
Servings: 4

Ingredients:

- 1 pound chicken thighs, boneless and skinless
- 1 tablespoon avocado oil
- 2 tablespoons mustard
- 1 shallot, chopped
- 1 cup chicken stock
- A pinch of salt and black pepper
- 3 garlic cloves, minced
- ½ teaspoon basil, dried

Directions:

1. Heat up a pan with the oil over medium heat, add the shallot, garlic and the chicken and brown everything for 5 minutes.
2. Add the mustard and the rest of the ingredients, toss gently, bring to a simmer and cook over medium heat for 30 minutes.
3. Divide everything between plates and serve hot.

Nutrition info per serving: calories 299, fat 15.5, fiber 6.6, carbs 30.3, protein 12.5

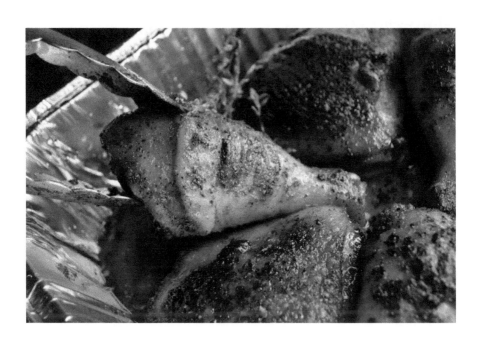

Chicken and Celery Mix

Prep time: 10 minutes I **Cooking time:** 35 minutes I
Servings: 4

Ingredients:

- A pinch of black pepper
- 2 pounds chicken breast, skinless, boneless and cubed
- 2 tablespoons olive oil
- 1 cup celery, chopped
- 3 garlic cloves, minced
- 1 poblano pepper, chopped
- 1 cup veggie stock
- 1 teaspoon chili powder
- 2 tablespoons chives, chopped

Directions:

1. Heat up a pan with the oil over medium heat, add the garlic, celery and poblano pepper, toss and cook for 5 minutes.
2. Add the meat, toss and cook for another 5 minutes.

3. Add the rest of the ingredients except the chives, bring to a simmer and cook over medium heat for 25 minutes more.
4. Divide the whole mix between plates and serve with the chives sprinkled on top.

Nutrition info per serving: calories 305, fat 18, fiber 13.4, carbs 22.5, protein 6

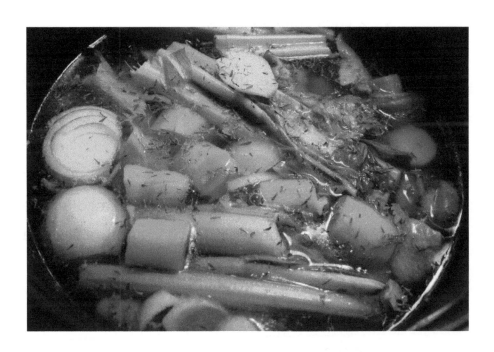

Lime Turkey

Prep time: 10 minutes I **Cooking time:** 40 minutes I
Servings: 4

Ingredients:

- 1 turkey breast, skinless, boneless and sliced
- 2 tablespoons olive oil
- 1 pound baby potatoes, peeled and halved
- 1 tablespoon sweet paprika
- 1 yellow onion, chopped
- 1 teaspoon chili powder
- 1 teaspoon rosemary, dried
- 2 cups chicken stock
- A pinch of black pepper
- Zest of 1 lime, grated
- 1 tablespoon lime juice
- 1 tablespoon cilantro, chopped

Directions:

1. Heat up a pan with the oil over medium heat, add the onion, chili powder and the rosemary, toss and sauté for 5 minutes.
2. Add the meat, and brown for 5 minutes more.
3. Add the potatoes and the rest of the ingredients except the cilantro, toss gently, bring to a

14

simmer and cook over medium heat for 30 minutes.

4. Divide the mix between plates and serve with the cilantro sprinkled on top.

Nutrition info per serving: calories 345, fat 22.2, fiber 12.3, carbs 34.5, protein 16.4

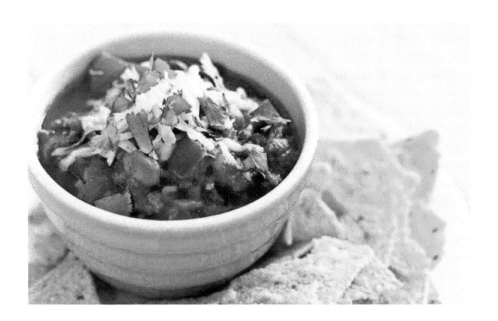

Chicken with Balsamic Mustard Greens

Prep time: 10 minutes I **Cooking time:** 25 minutes I
Servings: 4

Ingredients:

- 2 chicken breasts, skinless, boneless and cubed
- 3 cups mustard greens
- 1 cup tomatoes, chopped
- 1 red onion, chopped
- 2 tablespoons avocado oil
- 1 teaspoon oregano, dried
- 2 garlic cloves, minced
- 1 tablespoon chives, chopped
- 1 tablespoon balsamic vinegar
- A pinch of black pepper

Directions:

1. Heat up a pan with the oil over medium-high heat, add the onion and the garlic and sauté for 5 minutes.
2. Add the meat and brown it for 5 minutes more.
3. Add the greens, tomatoes and the other ingredients, toss, cook for 20 minutes over medium heat, divide between plates and serve.

Nutrition info per serving: calories 290, fat 12.3, fiber 6.7, carbs 22.30, protein 14.3

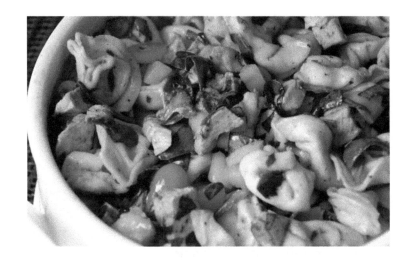

Baked Chicken

Prep time: 10 minutes I **Cooking time:** 50 minutes I
Servings: 4

Ingredients:

- 2 pounds chicken thighs, boneless and skinless
- 2 tablespoons olive oil
- 2 red onions, sliced
- A pinch of black pepper
- 1 teaspoon thyme, dried
- 1 teaspoon basil, dried
- 1 cup green apples, cored and roughly cubed
- 2 garlic cloves, minced
- 2 cups chicken stock
- 1 tablespoon lemon juice
- 1 cup tomatoes, cubed
- 1 tablespoon cilantro, chopped

Directions:

1. Heat up a pan with the oil over medium-high heat, add the onions and garlic, and sauté for 5 minutes.
2. Add the chicken and brown for another 5 minutes.
3. Add the thyme, basil and the other ingredients, toss gently, introduce in the oven and bake at 390 degrees F for 40 minutes.
4. Divide the chicken and apples mix between plates and serve.

Nutrition info per serving: calories 290, fat 12.3, fiber 4, carbs 15.7, protein 10

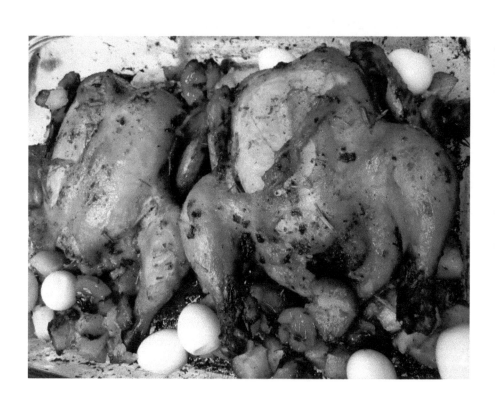

Chipotle Chicken

Prep time: 10 minutes I **Cooking time:** 1 hour I
Servings: 6

Ingredients:

- 2 pounds chicken thighs, boneless and skinless
- 1 yellow onion, chopped
- 2 tablespoons olive oil
- 3 garlic cloves, minced
- 1 tablespoon coriander seeds, ground
- 1 teaspoon cumin, ground
- 1 cup chicken stock
- 4 tablespoons chipotle chili paste
- A pinch of black pepper
- 1 tablespoon coriander, chopped

Directions:

1. Heat up a pan with the oil over medium heat, add the onion and the garlic and sauté for 5 minutes.
2. Add the meat and brown for 5 minutes more.
3. Add the rest of the ingredients, toss, introduce everything in the oven and bake at 390 degrees F for 50 minutes.
4. Divide the whole mix between plates and serve.

Nutrition info per serving: calories 280, fat 12.1, fiber 6.3, carbs 15.7, protein 12

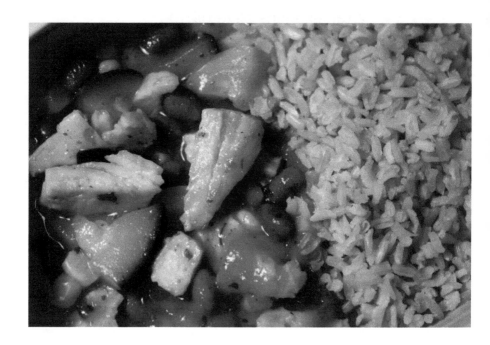

Mixed Herbed Turkey

Prep time: 10 minutes I **Cooking time:** 35 minutes I
Servings: 4

Ingredients:

- 1 big turkey breast, boneless, skinless and sliced
- 1 tablespoon chives, chopped
- 1 tablespoon oregano, chopped
- 1 tablespoon basil, chopped
- 1 tablespoon coriander, chopped
- 2 shallots, chopped
- 2 tablespoons olive oil
- 1 cup chicken stock
- 1 cup tomatoes, cubed
- Salt and black pepper to the taste

Directions:

1. Heat up a pan with the oil over medium heat, add the shallots and the meat and brown for 5 minutes.
2. Add the chives and the other ingredients, toss, bring to a simmer and cook over medium heat for 30 minutes.
3. Divide the mix between plates and serve.

Nutrition info per serving: calories 290, fat 11.9, fiber 5.5, carbs 16.2, protein 9

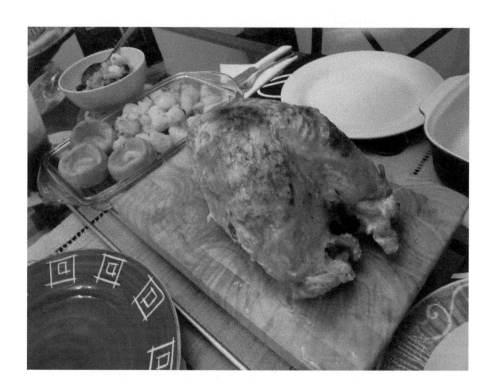

Chicken and Balsamic Ginger Sauce

Prep time: 10 minutes I **Cooking time:** 35 minutes I
Servings: 4

Ingredients:

- 1 pound chicken breast, skinless, boneless and cubed
- 1 tablespoon ginger, grated
- 1 tablespoon olive oil
- 2 shallots, chopped
- 1 tablespoon balsamic vinegar
- A pinch of black pepper
- ¾ cup chicken stock
- 1 tablespoon basil, chopped

Directions:

1. Heat up a pan with the oil over medium heat, add the shallots and the ginger, stir and sauté for 5 minutes.
2. Add the rest of the ingredients except the chicken, toss, bring to a simmer and cook for 5 minutes more.
3. Add the chicken, toss, simmer the whole mix for 25 minutes, divide between plates and serve.

Nutrition info per serving: calories 294, fat 15.5, fiber 3, carbs 15.4, protein 13.1

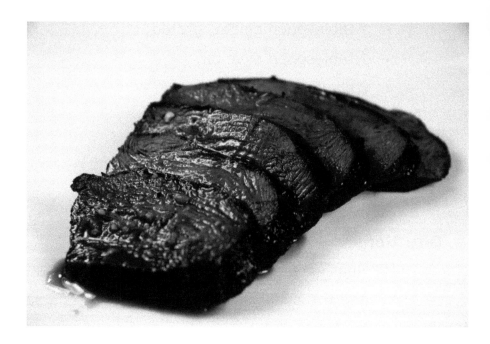

Chicken and Smoked Paprika Corn

Prep time: 10 minutes I **Cooking time:** 35 minutes I
Servings: 4

Ingredients:

- 2 pounds chicken breast, skinless, boneless and halved
- 2 cups corn
- 2 tablespoons avocado oil
- A pinch of black pepper
- 1 teaspoon smoked paprika
- 1 bunch green onions, chopped
- 1 cup chicken stock

Directions:

1. Heat up a pan with the oil over medium-high heat, add the green onions, stir and sauté them for 5 minutes.
2. Add the chicken and brown it for 5 minutes more.
3. Add the corn and the other ingredients, toss, introduce the pan in the oven and cook at 390 degrees F for 25 minutes.
4. Divide the mix between plates and serve.

Nutrition info per serving: calories 270, fat 12.4, fiber 5.2, carbs 12, protein 9

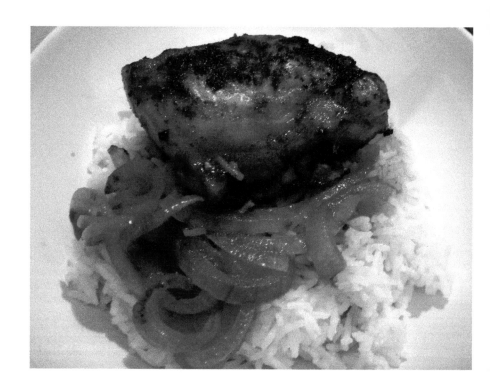

Curry Turkey and Lime Quinoa

Prep time: 10 minutes I **Cooking time:** 40 minutes I
Servings: 4

Ingredients:

- 1 pound turkey breast, skinless, boneless and cubed
- 1 tablespoon olive oil
- 1 cup quinoa
- 2 cups chicken stock
- 1 tablespoon lime juice
- 1 tablespoon parsley, chopped
- A pinch of black pepper
- 1 tablespoon red curry paste

Directions:

1. Heat up a pan with the oil over medium-high heat, add the meat and brown it for 5 minutes.
2. Add the quinoa and the rest of the ingredients, toss, bring to a simmer and cook over medium heat for 35 minutes.
3. Divide everything between plates and serve.

Nutrition info per serving: calories 310, fat 8.5, fiber 11, carbs 30.4, protein 16.3

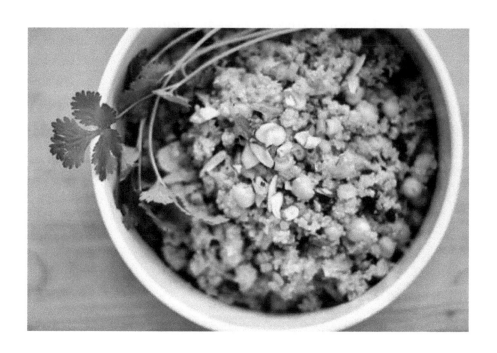

Turkey and Parsnips

Prep time: 10 minutes I **Cooking time:** 40 minutes I
Servings: 4

Ingredients:

- 1 pound turkey breast, skinless, boneless and cubed
- 2 parsnips, peeled and cubed
- 2 teaspoons cumin, ground
- 1 tablespoon parsley, chopped
- 2 tablespoons avocado oil
- 2 shallots, chopped
- 1 cup chicken stock
- 4 garlic cloves, minced
- A pinch of black pepper

Directions:

1. Heat up a pan with the oil over medium heat, add the shallots and the garlic and sauté for 5 minutes.
2. Add the turkey, toss and cook for 5 minutes more.

3. Add the parsnips and the other ingredients, toss, simmer over medium heat for 30 minutes more, divide between plates and serve.

Nutrition info per serving: calories 284, fat 18.2, fiber 4, carbs 16.7, protein 12.3

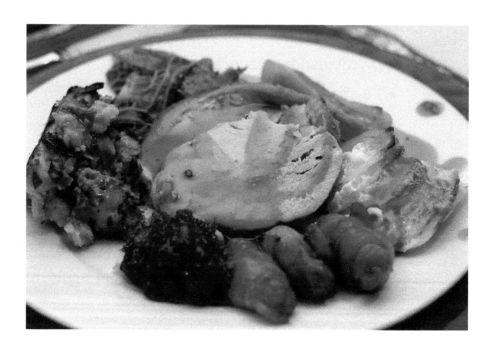

Turkey and Cilantro Lentils

Prep time: 10 minutes I **Cooking time:** 40 minutes I
Servings: 4

Ingredients:

- 1 cup lentils, cooked
- 1 cup chicken stock
- 1 pound turkey breast, skinless, boneless and cubed
- A pinch of black pepper
- 1 teaspoon oregano, dried
- 1 teaspoon nutmeg, ground
- 2 tablespoons olive oil
- 1 yellow onion, chopped
- 1 green bell pepper, chopped
- 1 cup cilantro, chopped

Directions:

1. Heat up a pan with the oil over medium heat, add the onion, bell pepper and the meat and cook for 10 minutes stirring often.
2. Add the rest of the ingredients, toss, bring to a simmer and cook over medium heat for 30 minutes.
3. Divide the mix between plates and serve.

Nutrition info per serving: calories 304, fat 11.2, fiber 4.5, carbs 22.2, protein 17

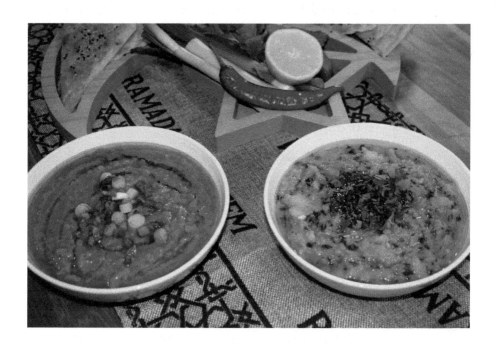

Turkey and Masala Rice

Prep time: 10 minutes I **Cooking time:** 40 minutes I
Servings: 4

Ingredients:

- 2 pounds turkey breast, skinless, boneless and cubed
- 1 cup brown rice
- 1 tablespoon green curry paste
- 1 teaspoon garam masala
- 2 tablespoons olive oil
- 1 yellow onion, chopped
- 1 garlic clove, minced
- A pinch of black pepper
- 1 tablespoon cilantro, chopped

Directions:

1. Heat up a pan with the oil over medium heat, add the onion, garlic and the meat and brown for 5 minutes stirring often.
2. Add the rice and the other ingredients, bring to a simmer and cook over medium heat for 35 minutes.
3. Divide the mix between plates and serve.

Nutrition info per serving: calories 489, fat 12.1, fiber 16.4, carbs 42.4, protein 51.5

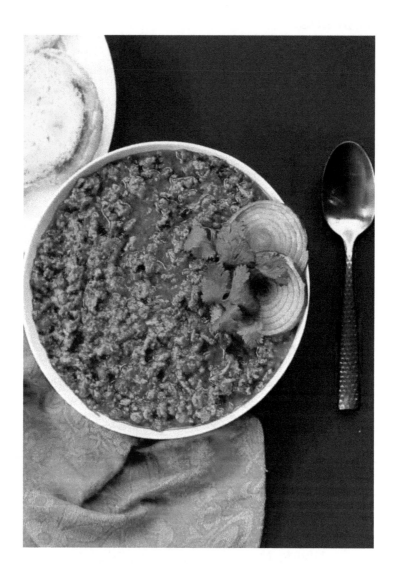

Turkey with Cilantro Beans and Olives

Prep time: 10 minutes I **Cooking time:** 35 minutes I

Servings: 4

Ingredients:

- 1 cup black beans, cooked
- 1 cup green olives, pitted and halved
- 1 pound turkey breast, skinless, boneless and sliced
- 1 tablespoon cilantro, chopped
- 1 cup tomato passata
- 1 tablespoon olive oil

Directions:

1. Grease a baking dish with the oil, arrange the turkey slices inside, add the other ingredients as well, introduce in the oven and bake at 380 degrees F for 35 minutes.
2. Divide between plates and serve.

Nutrition info per serving: calories 331, fat 6.4, fiber 9, carbs 38.5, protein 30.7

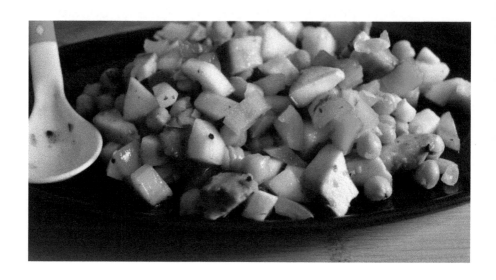

Chicken and Tomato Quinoa

Prep time: 10 minutes I **Cooking time:** 35 minutes I
Servings: 8

Ingredients:

- 1 tablespoon olive oil
- 2 pounds chicken breasts, skinless, boneless and halved
- 1 teaspoon rosemary, ground
- A pinch of salt and black pepper
- 2 shallots, chopped
- 1 tablespoon olive oil
- 3 tablespoons tomato passata
- 2 cups quinoa, already cooked

Directions:

1. Heat up a pan with the oil over medium-high heat, add the meat and shallots and brown for 2 minutes on each side.
2. Add the rosemary and the other ingredients, toss, introduce in the oven and cook at 370 degrees F for 30 minutes.
3. Divide the mix between plates and serve.

Nutrition info per serving: calories 406, fat 14.5, fiber 3.1, carbs 28.1, protein 39

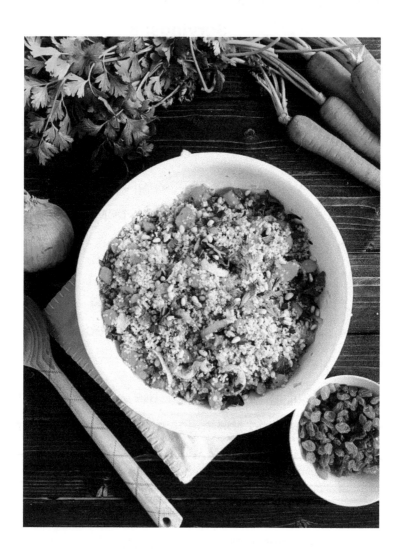

Garlic Chicken Wings

Prep time: 10 minutes I **Cooking time:** 20 minutes I
Servings: 4

Ingredients:

- 2 pounds chicken wings
- 2 teaspoons allspice, ground
- 2 tablespoons avocado oil
- 5 garlic cloves, minced
- Black pepper to the taste
- 2 tablespoons chives, chopped

Directions:

1. In a bowl, combine the chicken wings with the allspice and the other ingredients and toss well.
2. Arrange the chicken wings in a roasting pan and bake at 400 degrees F for 20 minutes.
3. Divide the chicken wings between plates and serve.

Nutrition info per serving: calories 449, fat 17.8, fiber 0.6, carbs 2.4, protein 66.1

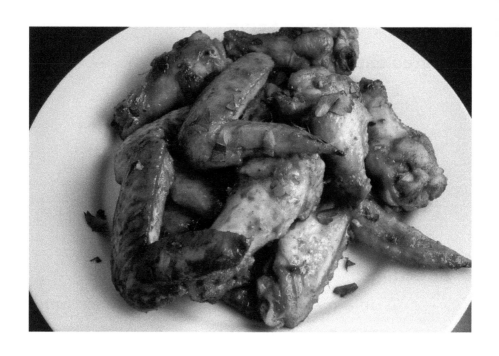

Parsley Chicken and Snow Peas

Prep time: 10 minutes I **Cooking time:** 30 minutes I
Servings: 4

Ingredients:

- 2 pounds chicken breasts, skinless, boneless and cubed
- 2 cups snow peas
- 2 tablespoons olive oil
- 1 red onion, chopped
- 1 cup tomato passata
- 2 tablespoons parsley, chopped
- A pinch of black pepper

Directions:

1. Heat up a pan with the oil over medium heat, add the onion and the meat and brown for 5 minutes.
2. Add the peas and the rest of the ingredients, bring to a simmer and cook over medium heat for 25 minutes.
3. Divide the mix between plates and serve.

Nutrition info per serving: calories 551, fat 24.2, fiber 3.8, carbs 11.7, protein 69.4

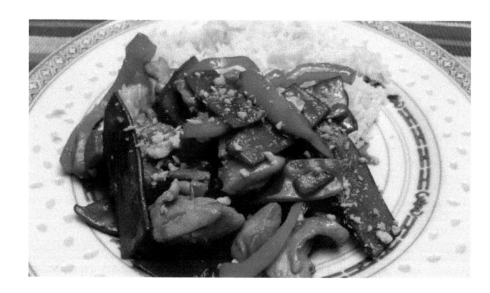

Turkey and Cilantro Broccoli

Prep time: 10 minutes I **Cooking time:** 30 minutes I
Servings: 4

Ingredients:
- 1 red onion, chopped
- 1 pound turkey breast, skinless, boneless and cubed
- 2 cups broccoli florets
- 1 teaspoon cumin, ground
- 3 garlic cloves, minced
- 2 tablespoons olive oil
- 14 ounces coconut milk
- A pinch of black pepper
- ¼ cup cilantro, chopped

Directions:
1. Heat up a pot with the oil over medium heat, add the onion and the garlic, stir and sauté for 5 minutes.
2. Add the turkey, toss and brown for 5 minutes.
3. Add the broccoli and the rest of the ingredients, bring to a simmer over medium heat and cook for 20 minutes.

45

4. Divide the mix between plates and serve.

Nutrition info per serving: calories 438, fat 32.9, fiber 4.7, carbs 16.8, protein 23.5

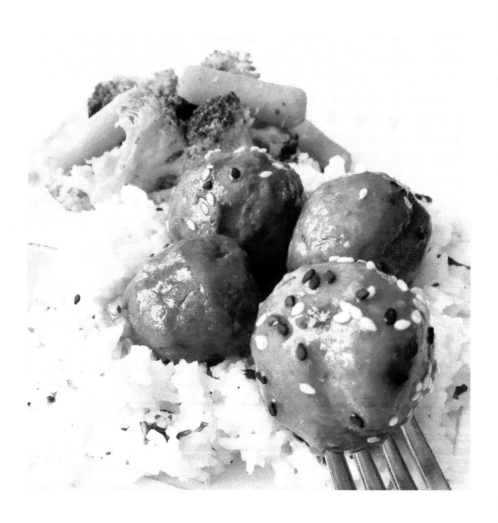

Cloves Chicken

Prep time: 10 minutes I **Cooking time:** 30 minutes I
Servings: 4

Ingredients:

- 1 pound chicken breast, skinless, boneless and cubed
- 1 cup chicken stock
- 1 tablespoons avocado oil
- 2 teaspoons cloves, ground
- 1 yellow onion, chopped
- 2 teaspoons sweet paprika
- 3 tomatoes, cubed
- A pinch of salt and black pepper
- ½ cup parsley, chopped

Directions:

1. Heat up a pan with the oil over medium heat, add the onion and sauté for 5 minutes.
2. Add the chicken and brown for 5 minutes more.
3. Add the stock and the rest of the ingredients, bring to a simmer and cook over medium heat for 20 minutes more.
4. Divide the mix between plates and serve.

Nutrition info per serving: calories 324, fat 12.3, fiber 5, carbs 33.10, protein 22.4

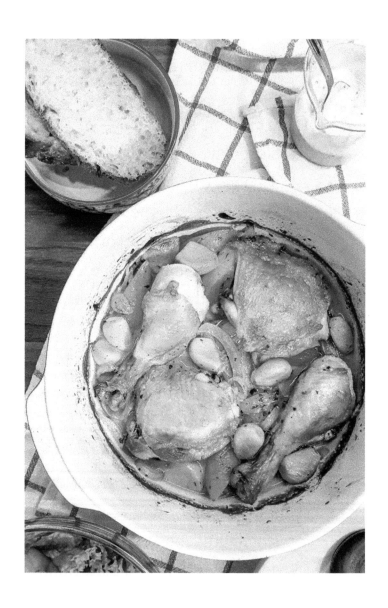

Chicken with Ginger

Prep time: 10 minutes I **Cooking time:** 30 minutes I
Servings: 4

Ingredients:

- 2 chicken breasts, skinless, boneless and halved
- 1 tablespoon ginger, grated
- 1 cup tomatoes, chopped
- 2 tablespoons lemon juice
- 2 tablespoons olive oil
- A pinch of black pepper

Directions:

1. Heat up a pan with the oil over medium heat, add the ginger, toss and cook for 5 minutes.
2. Add the chicken and cook for 5 minutes more.
3. Add the rest of the ingredients, bring to a simmer and cook for 20 minutes more.
4. Divide everything between plates and serve.

Nutrition info per serving: calories 300, fat 14.5, fiber 5.3, carbs 16.4, protein 15.1

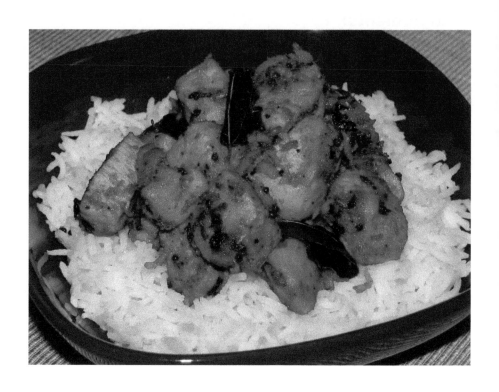

Garlic Turkey and Spring Onions

Prep time: 10 minutes I **Cooking time:** 30 minutes I
Servings: 4

Ingredients:

- ½ tablespoon black peppercorns
- 1 tablespoon olive oil
- 1 pound turkey breast, skinless, boneless and cubed
- 1 cup chicken stock
- 3 garlic cloves, minced
- 2 tomatoes, cubed
- A pinch of black pepper
- 2 tablespoons spring onions, chopped

Directions:

1. Heat up a pan with the oil over medium heat, add the garlic and the turkey and brown for 5 minutes.
2. Add the peppercorns and the rest of the ingredients, bring to a simmer and cook over medium heat for 25 minutes.
3. Divide the mix between plates and serve.

Nutrition info per serving: calories 313, fat 13.3, fiber 7, carbs 23.4, protein 16

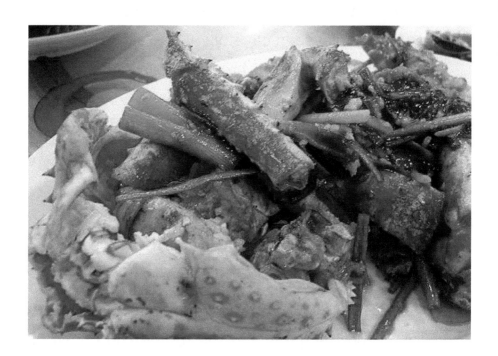

Chicken and Rosemary Veggies

Prep time: 10 minutes I **Cooking time:** 40 minutes I
Servings: 4

Ingredients:

- 2 pounds chicken breasts, skinless, boneless and cubed
- 1 carrot, cubed
- 1 celery stalk, chopped
- 1 tomato, cubed
- 2 small red onions, sliced
- 1 zucchini, cubed
- 2 garlic cloves, minced
- 1 tablespoon rosemary, chopped
- 2 tablespoons olive oil
- Black pepper to the taste
- ½ cup veggie stock

Directions:

1. Heat up a pan with the oil over medium heat, add the onions and the garlic, stir and sauté for 5 minutes.
2. Add the chicken, toss and brown it for 5 minutes more.
3. Add the carrot and the other ingredients, toss, bring to a simmer and cook over medium heat for 30 minutes.
4. Divide the mix between plates and serve.

Nutrition info per serving: calories 325, fat 22.5, fiber 6.1, carbs 15.5, protein 33.2

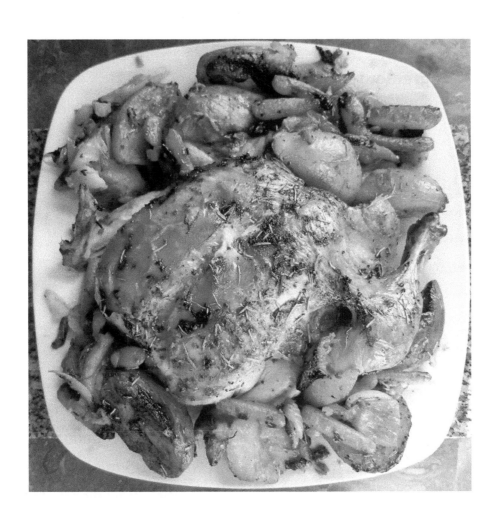

Chicken with Carrots

Prep time: 10 minutes I **Cooking time:** 25 minutes I
Servings: 4

Ingredients:

- 1 pound chicken breast, skinless, boneless and cubed
- 2 tablespoons olive oil
- 2 carrots, peeled and grated
- 1 teaspoon sweet paprika
- ½ cup veggie stock
- 1 red cabbage head, shredded
- 1 yellow onion, chopped
- Black pepper to the taste

Directions:

1. Heat up a pan with the oil over medium heat, add the onion, stir and sauté for 5 minutes.
2. Add the meat, and brown it for 5 minutes more.
3. Add the carrots and the other ingredients, toss, bring to a simmer and cook over medium heat for 15 minutes.
4. Divide everything between plates and serve.

Nutrition info per serving: calories 370, fat 22.2, fiber 5.2, carbs 44.2, protein 24.2

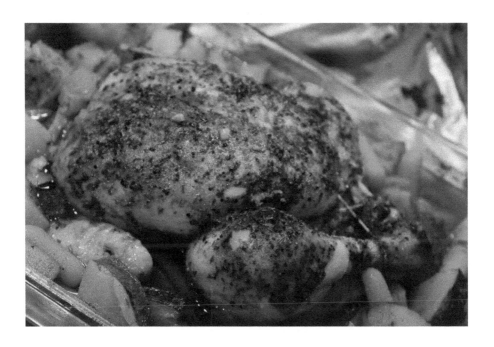

Turkey Sandwich

Prep time: 10 minutes I **Cooking time:** 25 minutes I
Servings: 4

Ingredients:

- 1 turkey breast, skinless, boneless and sliced into 4 pieces
- 1 eggplant, sliced into 4 slices
- Black pepper to the taste
- 1 tablespoon olive oil
- 1 tablespoon oregano, chopped
- ½ cup tomato sauce
- ½ cup cheddar cheese, shredded
- 4 whole wheat bread slices

Directions:

1. Heat up a grill over medium-high heat, add the turkey slices, drizzle half of the oil over them, sprinkle the black pepper, cook for 8 minutes on each side and transfer to a plate.

2. Arrange the eggplant slices on the heated grill, drizzle the rest of the oil over them, season with black pepper as well, cook them for 4 minutes on each side and transfer to the plate with the turkey slices as well.

3. Arrange 2 bread slices on a working surface, divide the cheese on each, divide the eggplant slices and turkey ones on each, sprinkle the oregano, drizzle the sauce all over and top with the other 2 bread slices.

4. Divide the sandwiches between plates and serve.

Nutrition info per serving: calories 280, fat 12.2, fiber 6, carbs 14, protein 12

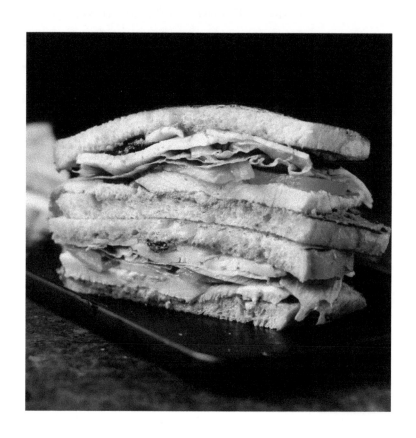

Turkey Tortillas

Prep time: 10 minutes I **Cooking time:** 20 minutes I
Servings: 4

Ingredients:

- 4 whole wheat tortillas
- ½ cup yogurt
- 1 pound turkey, breast, skinless, boneless and cut into strips
- 1 tablespoon olive oil
- 1 red onion, sliced
- 1 zucchini, cubed
- 2 tomatoes, cubed
- Black pepper to the taste

Directions:

1. Heat up a pan with the oil over medium heat, add the onion, stir and sauté for 5 minutes.
2. Add the zucchini and tomatoes, toss and cook for 2 minutes more.
3. Add the turkey meat, toss and cook for 13 minutes more.

4. Spread the yogurt on each tortilla, add divide the turkey and zucchini mix, roll, divide between plates and serve.

Nutrition info per serving: calories 290, fat 13.4, fiber 3.42, carbs 12.5, protein 6.9

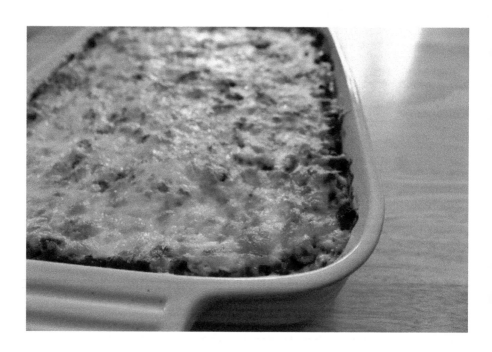

Chicken with Coconut Veggies

Prep time: 10 minutes I **Cooking time:** 25 minutes I
Servings: 4

Ingredients:

- 2 chicken breasts, skinless, boneless and cubed
- 1 red onion, chopped
- 2 tablespoons olive oil
- 1 eggplant, cubed
- 1 red bell pepper, cubed
- 1 yellow bell pepper, cubed
- Black pepper to the taste
- 2 cups coconut milk

Directions:

1. Heat up a pan with the oil over medium-high heat, add the onion, stir and cook for 3 minutes.
2. Add the bell peppers, toss and cook for 2 minutes more.
3. Add the chicken and the other ingredients, toss, bring to a simmer and cook over medium heat for 20 minutes more.
4. Divide everything between plates and serve.

Nutrition info per serving: calories 310, fat 14.7, fiber 4, carbs 14.5, protein 12.6

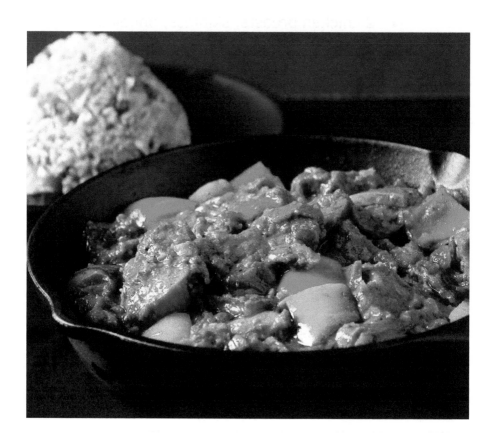

Balsamic Italian Turkey

Prep time: 10 minutes I **Cooking time:** 40 minutes I
Servings: 4

Ingredients:

- 1 big turkey breast, skinless, boneless and sliced
- 2 tablespoons balsamic vinegar
- 1 tablespoon olive oil
- 2 garlic cloves, minced
- 1 tablespoon Italian seasoning
- Black pepper to the taste
- 1 tablespoon cilantro, chopped

Directions:

1. In a baking dish, mix the turkey with the vinegar, the oil and the other ingredients, toss, introduce in the oven at 400 degrees F and bake for 40 minutes.
2. Divide everything between plates and serve with a side salad.

Nutrition info per serving: calories 280, fat 12.7, fiber 3, carbs 22.1, protein 14

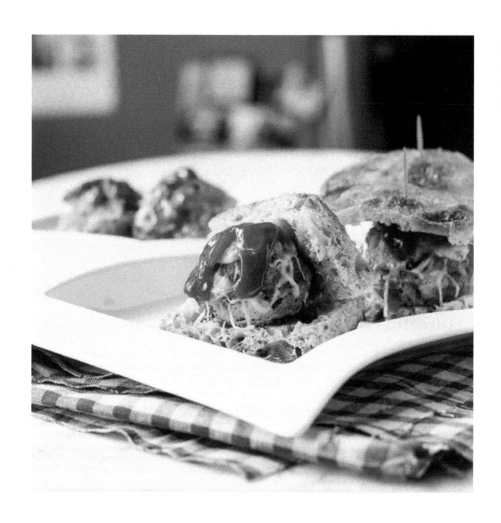

Cheddar Turkey

Prep time: 10 minutes I **Cooking time:** 1 hour I
Servings: 4

Ingredients:

- 1 pound turkey breast, skinless, boneless and sliced
- 2 tablespoons olive oil
- 1 cup tomatoes, chopped
- Black pepper to the taste
- 1 cup cheddar cheese, shredded
- 2 tablespoons parsley, chopped

Directions:

1. Grease a baking dish with the oil, arrange the turkey slices into the pan, spread the tomatoes over them, season with black pepper, sprinkle the cheese and parsley on top, introduce in the oven at 400 degrees F and bake for 1 hour.
2. Divide everything between plates and serve.

Nutrition info per serving: calories 350, fat 13.1, fiber 4, carbs 32.4, protein 14.65

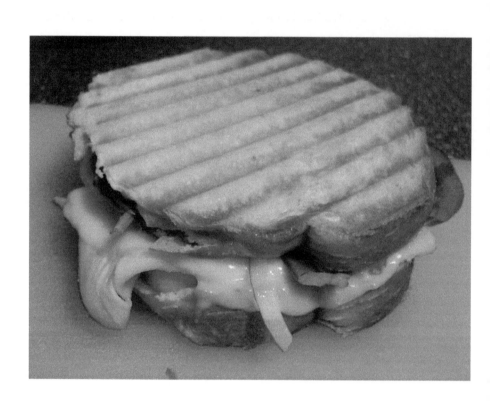

Coconut Parmesan Turkey

Prep time: 10 minutes I **Cooking time:** 23 minutes I
Servings: 4

Ingredients:

- 1 pound turkey breast, skinless, boneless and cubed
- 1 tablespoon olive oil
- ½ cup parmesan, grated
- 2 shallots, chopped
- 1 cup coconut milk
- Black pepper to the taste

Directions:

1. Heat up a pan with the oil over medium-high heat, add the shallots, toss and cook for 5 minutes.
2. Add the meat, coconut milk, and black pepper, toss and cook over medium heat for 15 minutes more.
3. Add the parmesan, cook for 2-3 minutes, divide everything between plates and serve.

Nutrition info per serving: calories 320, fat 11.4, fiber 3.5, carbs 14.3, protein 11.3

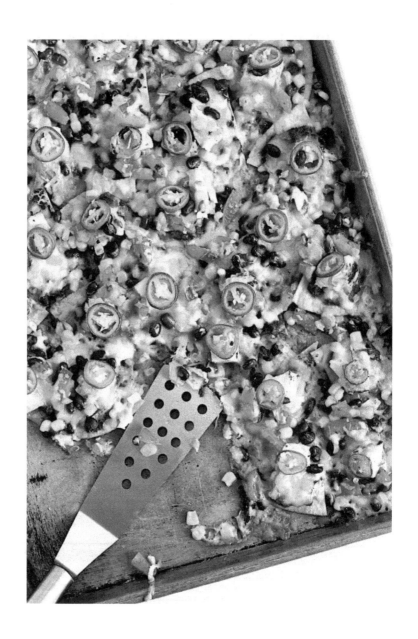

Chicken and Shrimp Mix

Prep time: 10 minutes I **Cooking time:** 14 minutes I
Servings: 4

Ingredients:

- 1 tablespoon olive oil
- 1 pound chicken breast, skinless, boneless and cubed
- ¼ cup chicken stock
- 1 pound shrimp, peeled and deveined
- ½ cup coconut cream
- 1 tablespoon cilantro, chopped

Directions:

1. Heat up a pan with the oil over medium heat, add the chicken, toss and cook for 8 minutes.
2. Add the shrimp and the other ingredients, toss, cook everything for 6 minutes more, divide into bowls and serve.

Nutrition info per serving: calories 370, fat 12.3, fiber 5.2, carbs 12.6, protein 8

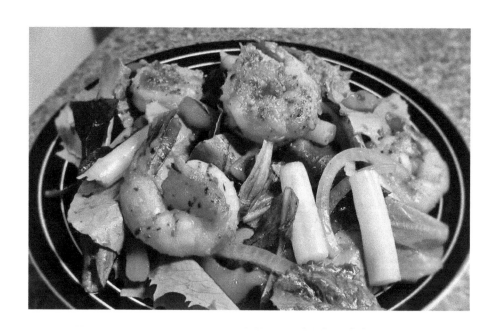

Basil Turkey

Prep time: 10 minutes I **Cooking time:** 40 minutes I
Servings: 4

Ingredients:

- 1 pound turkey breast, skinless, and cut into strips
- 1 cup coconut cream
- 1 cup chicken stock
- 2 tablespoons parsley, chopped
- 1 bunch asparagus, trimmed and halved
- 1 teaspoon chili powder
- 2 tablespoons olive oil
- A pinch of sea salt and black pepper

Directions:

1. Heat up a pan with the oil over medium-high heat, add the turkey and some black pepper, toss and cook for 5 minutes.
2. Add the asparagus, chili powder and the other ingredients, toss, bring to a simmer and cook over medium heat for 30 minutes more.
3. Divide everything between plates and serve.

Nutrition info per serving: calories 290, fat 12.10, fiber 4.6, carbs 12.7, protein 24

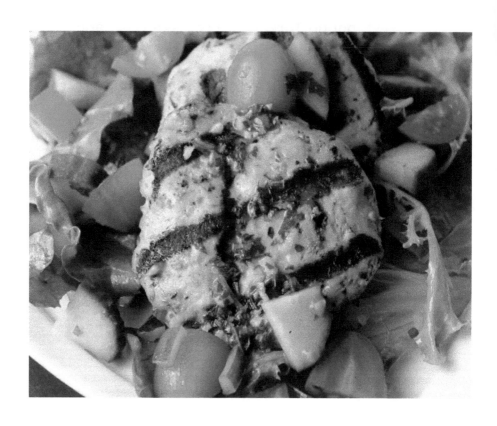

Cashew Turkey

Prep time: 10 minutes I **Cooking time:** 40 minutes I
Servings: 4

Ingredients:

- 1 pound turkey breast, skinless, boneless and cubed
- 1 cup cashews, chopped
- 1 yellow onion, chopped
- ½ tablespoon olive oil
- Black pepper to the taste
- ½ teaspoon sweet paprika
- 2 and ½ tablespoons cashew butter
- ¼ cup chicken stock
- 1 tablespoon cilantro, chopped

Directions:

1. Heat up a pan with the oil over medium-high heat, add the onion, stir and sauté for 5 minutes.
2. Add the meat and brown it for 5 minutes more.
3. Add the rest of the ingredients, toss, bring to a simmer and cook over medium heat for 30 minutes.

4. Divide the whole mix between plates and serve.

Nutrition info per serving: calories 352, fat 12.7, fiber 6.2, carbs 33.2, protein 13.5

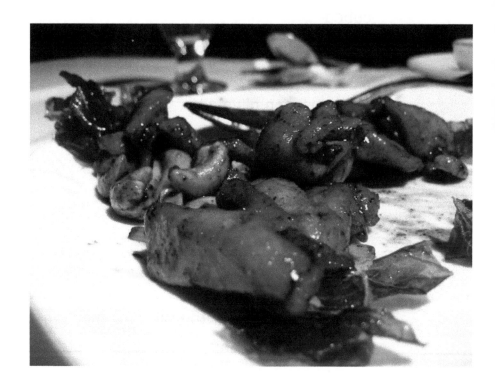

Turkey and Mango

Prep time: 10 minutes I **Cooking time:** 35 minutes I
Servings: 4

Ingredients:

- 2 pounds turkey breasts, skinless, boneless and cubed
- 1 tablespoon olive oil
- 1 red onion, chopped
- 1 cup mango, peeled and cubed
- 1 cup chicken stock
- ¼ cup cilantro, chopped
- Black pepper to the taste

Directions:

1. Heat up a pot with the oil over medium-high heat, add the onion, stir and sauté for 5 minutes.
2. Add the meat, berries and the other ingredients, bring to a simmer and cook over medium heat fro 30 minutes more.
3. Divide the mix between plates and serve.

Nutrition info per serving: calories 293, fat 7.3, fiber 2.8, carbs 14.7, protein 39.3

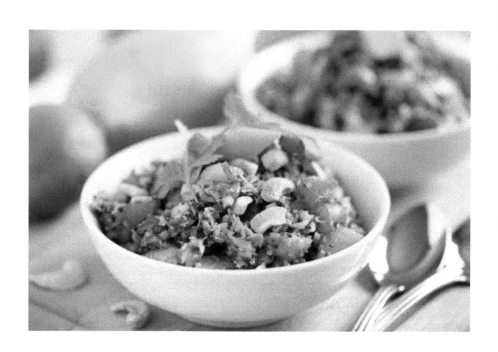

Five Spice Chicken

Prep time: 5 minutes I **Cooking time:** 35 minutes I
Servings: 4

Ingredients:

- 1 cup tomatoes, crushed
- 1 teaspoon five spice
- 2 chicken breast halves, skinless, boneless and halved
- 1 tablespoon avocado oil
- 2 tablespoons coconut aminos
- Black pepper to the taste
- 1 tablespoons hot pepper
- 1 tablespoon cilantro, chopped

Directions:

1. Heat up a pan with the oil over medium heat, add the meat and brown it for 2 minutes on each side.
2. Add the tomatoes, five spice and the other ingredients, bring to a simmer and cook over medium heat for 30 minutes.
3. Divide the whole mix between plates and serve.

Nutrition info per serving: calories 244, fat 8.4, fiber 1.1, carbs 4.5, protein 31

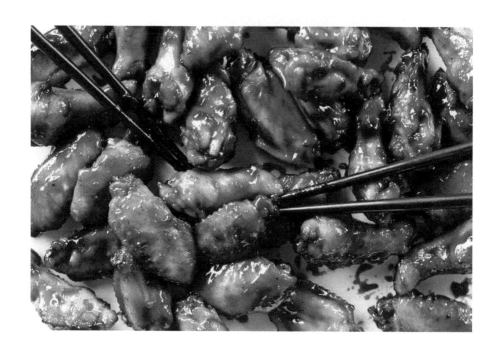

Turkey with Nutmeg Greens

Prep time: 10 minutes I **Cooking time:** 17 minutes I
Servings: 4

Ingredients:

- 1 pound turkey breast, boneless, skinless and cubed
- 1 cup mustard greens
- 1 teaspoon nutmeg, ground
- 1 teaspoon allspice, ground
- 1 yellow onion, chopped
- Black pepper to the taste
- 1 tablespoon olive oil

Directions:

1. Heat up a pan with the oil over medium-high heat, add the onion and the meat and brown for 5 minutes.
2. Add the rest of the ingredients, toss, cook over medium heat for 12 minutes more, divide between plates and serve.

Nutrition info per serving: calories 270, fat 8.4, fiber 8.32, carbs 33.3, protein 9

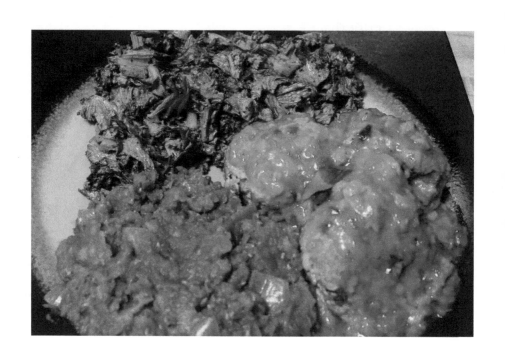

Chicken and Chili Tomato Mushroom Mix

Prep time: 10 minutes I **Cooking time:** 20 minutes I
Servings: 4

Ingredients:

- 2 chicken breasts, skinless, boneless and halved
- ½ pound white mushrooms, halved
- 1 tablespoon olive oil
- 1 cup tomatoes, chopped
- 2 tablespoons almonds, chopped
- 2 tablespoons olive oil
- ½ teaspoon chili flakes
- Black pepper to the taste

Directions:

1. Heat up a pan with the oil over medium-high heat, add the mushrooms, toss and sauté for 5 minutes.
2. Add the meat, toss and cook for 5 minutes more.
3. Add the tomatoes and the other ingredients, bring to a simmer and cook over medium heat for 10 minutes.

4. Divide the mix between plates and serve.

Nutrition info per serving: calories 320, fat 12.2, fiber 5.3, carbs 33.3, protein 15

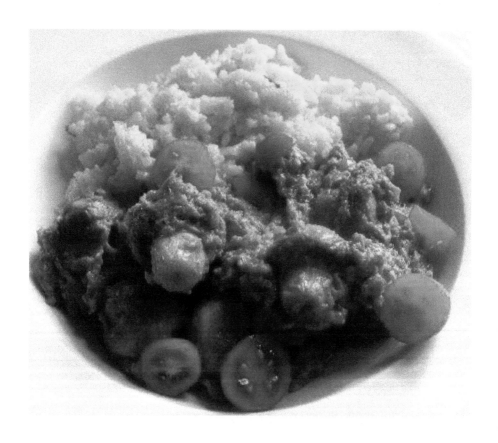

Chili Chicken and Pineapple

Prep time: 10 minutes

Cooking time: 20 minutes

Servings: 4

Ingredients:

- 2 red chilies, chopped
- 1 tablespoon olive oil
- 1 yellow onion, chopped
- 1 pound chicken breasts, skinless, boneless and cubed
- 1 cup tomatoes, crushed
- 2 cups pineapple, peeled and cubed
- Black pepper to the taste
- ½ cup chicken stock
- 2 tablespoons lime juice

Directions:

1. Heat up a pan with the oil over medium heat, add the onion and the chilies, stir and sauté for 5 minutes.
2. Add the meat, toss and brown for 5 minutes more.
3. Add the rest of the ingredients, bring to a simmer over medium heat and cook for 10 minutes.
4. Divide the mix between plates and serve.

Nutrition info per serving: calories 280, fat 11.3, fiber 5, carbs 14.5, protein 13.5

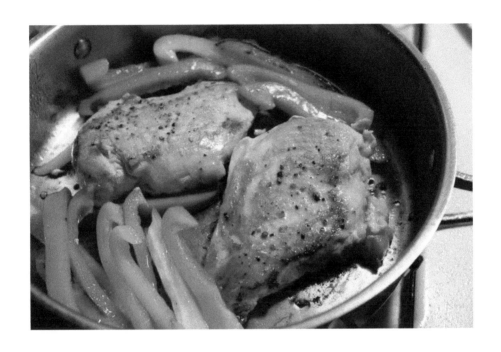

Chicken and Beets Mix

Prep time: 10 minutes I **Cooking time:** 0 minutes I
Servings: 4

Ingredients:

- 1 carrot, shredded
- 2 beets, peeled and shredded
- ½ cup avocado mayonnaise
- 1 cup smoked chicken breast, skinless, boneless, cooked and shredded
- 1 teaspoon chives, chopped

Directions:

1. In a bowl, combine the chicken with the beets and the other ingredients, toss and serve right away.

Nutrition info per serving: calories 288, fat 24.6, fiber 1.4, carbs 6.5, protein 14

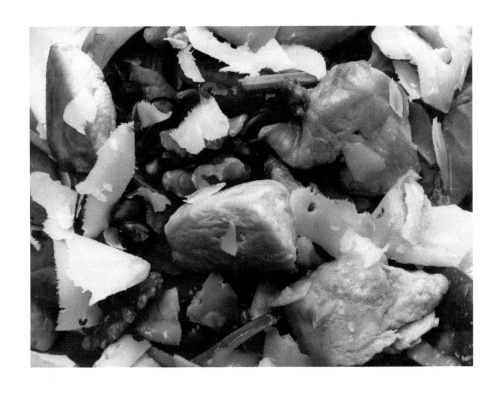

Turkey Salad

Prep time: 4 minutes I **Cooking time:** 0 minutes I
Servings: 4

Ingredients:

- 2 cups turkey breast, skinless, boneless, cooked and shredded
- 1 cup celery stalks, chopped
- 2 spring onions, chopped
- 1 cup black olives, pitted and halved
- 1 tablespoon olive oil
- 1 teaspoon lime juice
- 1 cup yogurt

Directions:

1. In a bowl, combine the turkey with the celery and the other ingredients, toss and serve cold.

Nutrition info per serving: calories 157, fat 8, fiber 2, carbs 10.8, protein 11.5

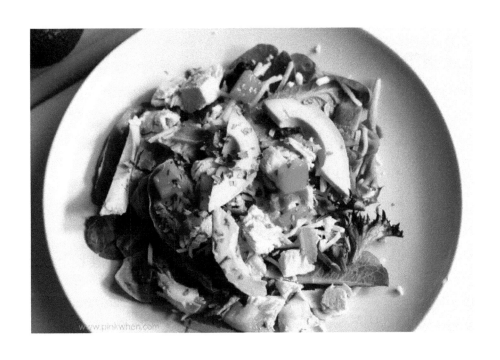

Chicken with Apples and Grapes Mix

Prep time: 10 minutes I **Cooking time:** 40 minutes I
Servings: 4

Ingredients:

- 1 apple, cubed
- 1 yellow onion, sliced
- 1 tablespoon olive oil
- 1 cup tomatoes, cubed
- ¼ cup chicken stock
- 2 garlic cloves, chopped
- 1 pound chicken thighs, skinless and boneless
- 1 cup green grapes
- Black pepper to the taste

Directions:

1. Grease a baking pan with the oil, arrange the chicken thighs inside and add the other ingredients on top.
2. Bake at 390 degrees F for 40 minutes, divide between plates and serve.

Nutrition info per serving: calories 289, fat 12.1, fiber 1.7, carbs 10.3, protein 33.9

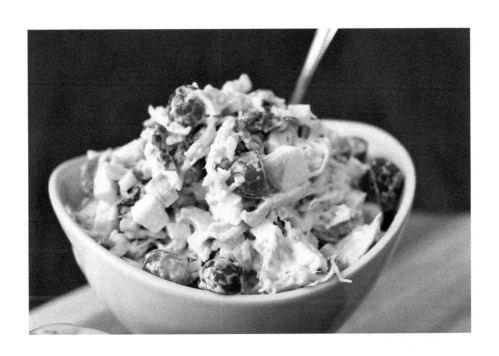

Turkey and Lemon Millet

Prep time: 5 minutes I **Cooking time:** 55 minutes I
Servings: 4

Ingredients:

- 1 tablespoon olive oil
- 1 turkey breast, skinless, boneless and sliced
- Black pepper to the taste
- 2 celery stalks, chopped
- 1 red onion, chopped
- 2 cups chicken stock
- ½ cup millet
- 1 teaspoon lemon zest, grated
- 1 tablespoon lemon juice
- 1 tablespoon chives, chopped

Directions:

1. Heat up a pot with the oil over medium-high heat, add the meat and the onion, toss and brown for 5 minutes.
2. Add the celery and the other ingredients, toss, bring to a simmer, reduce heat to medium, simmer for 50 minutes, divide into bowls and serve.

Nutrition info per serving: calories 150, fat 4.5, fiber 4.9, carbs 20.8, protein 7.5

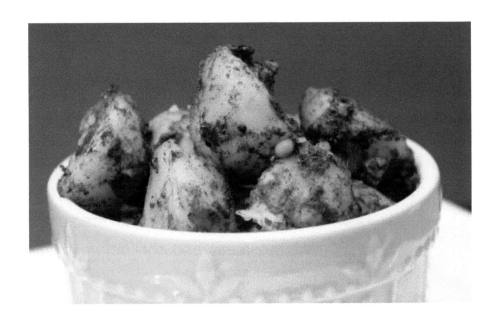

Turkey with Radish Mix

Prep time: 10 minutes I **Cooking time:** 35 minutes I
Servings: 4

Ingredients:

- 1 turkey breast, skinless, boneless and cubed
- 2 red beets, peeled and cubed
- 1 cup radishes, cubed
- 1 red onion, chopped
- ¼ cup chicken stock
- Black pepper to the taste
- 1 tablespoon olive oil
- 2 tablespoon chives, chopped

Directions:

1. Heat up a pan with the oil over medium-high heat, add the meat and the onion, toss and brown for 5 minutes.
2. Add the beets, radishes and the other ingredients, bring to a simmer and cook over medium heat for 30 minutes more.
3. Divide the mix between plates and serve.

Nutrition info per serving: calories 113, fat 4.4, fiber 2.3, carbs 10.4, protein 8.8

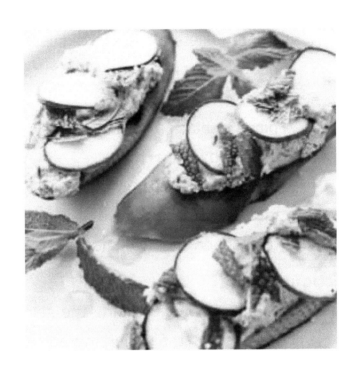

Salmon and Lemon Peaches Bowls

Prep time: 10 minutes I **Cooking time:** 0 minutes I
Servings: 4

Ingredients:

- 2 salmon fillets, boneless, skinless and cubed
- 2 peaches, stones removed and cubed
- 1 teaspoon olive oil
- A pinch of black pepper
- 2 cups baby spinach
- ½ tablespoon balsamic vinegar
- 1 tablespoon lemon juice
- 1 tablespoon cilantro, chopped

Directions:

1. In a salad bowl, combine the salmon with the peaches and the other ingredients, toss and serve cold.

Nutrition info per serving: calories 133, fat 7.1, fiber 1.5, carbs 8.2, protein 1.7

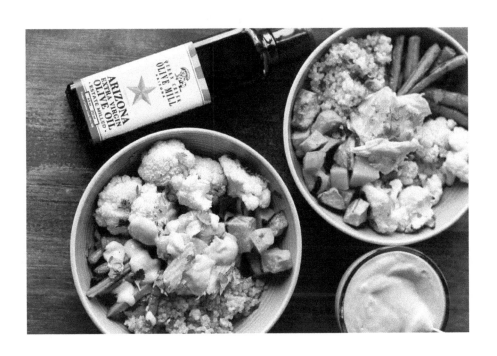

Coconut Salmon

Prep time: 10 minutes I **Cooking time:** 15 minutes I
Servings: 4

Ingredients:

- 2 tablespoons olive oil
- 4 salmon fillets, boneless
- 1 tablespoon capers, drained
- 1 tablespoon dill, chopped
- 1 shallot, chopped
- ½ cup coconut cream
- A pinch of black pepper

Directions:

1. Heat up a pan with the oil over medium-high heat, add the shallot and the capers, toss and sauté fro 4 minutes.
2. Add the salmon and cook it for 3 minutes on each side.
3. Add the rest of the ingredients, cook everything for 5 minutes more, divide between plates and serve.

Nutrition info per serving: calories 369, fat 25.2, fiber 0.9, carbs 2.7, protein 35.5

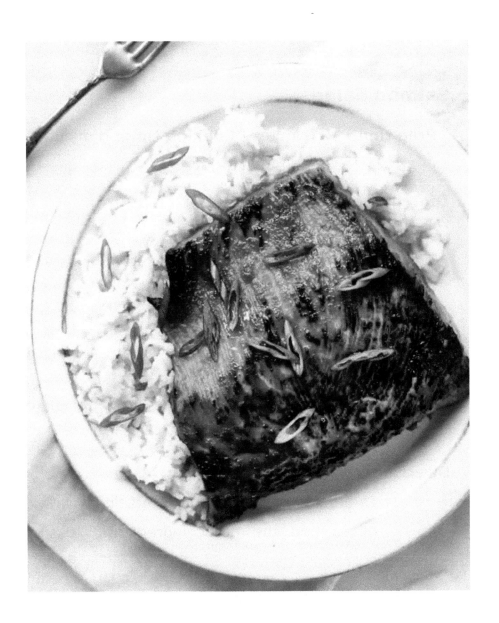

Salmon Salad

Prep time: 10 minutes I **Cooking time:** 0 minutes I
Servings: 4

Ingredients:

- 2 tablespoons olive oil
- ½ teaspoon lemon juice
- ½ teaspoon lemon zest, grated
- A pinch of black pepper
- 1 cup black olives, pitted and halved
- 1 cup cucumber, cubed
- ½ pound salmon, boiled, boneless and cubed
- 1 tablespoon chives, chopped

Directions:

1. In a salad bowl, combine the salmon with the olives and the other ingredients, toss and serve.

Nutrition info per serving: calories 170, fat 13.1, fiber 1.3, carbs 3.2, protein 10.9

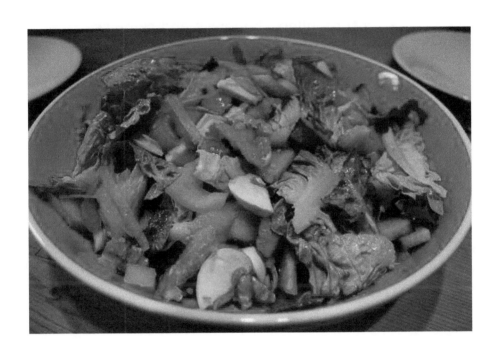

Lime Tuna Mix

Prep time: 10 minutes I **Cooking time:** 15 minutes I
Servings: 4

Ingredients:

- 4 tuna fillets, boneless and skinless
- 1 tablespoon olive oil
- 2 shallots, chopped
- 2 tablespoons lime juice
- A pinch of black pepper
- 1 teaspoon sweet paprika
- ½ cup chicken stock

Directions:

1. Heat up a pan with the oil over medium-high heat, add shallots and sauté for 3 minutes.
2. Add the fish and cook it for 4 minutes on each side.
3. Add the rest of the ingredients, cook everything for 3 minutes more, divide between plates and serve.

Nutrition info per serving: calories 404, fat 34.6, fiber 0.3, carbs 3, protein 21.4

Cod and Shallot Mix

Prep time: 10 minutes I **Cooking time:** 17 minutes I
Servings: 4

Ingredients:

- 2 tablespoons olive oil
- 1 tablespoon lemon juice
- 1 tablespoon mint, chopped
- 4 cod fillets, boneless
- 1 teaspoons lemon zest, grated
- A pinch of black pepper
- ¼ cup shallot, chopped
- ½ cup chicken stock

Directions:

1. Heat up a pan with the oil over medium heat, add the shallots, stir and sauté for 5 minutes.
2. Add the cod, the lemon juice and the other ingredients, bring to a simmer and cook over medium heat for 12 minutes.
3. Divide everything between plates and serve.

Nutrition info per serving: calories 160, fat 8.1, fiber 0.2, carbs 2, protein 20.5

Garlic Cod and Tomatoes

Prep time: 10 minutes I **Cooking time:** 16 minutes I
Servings: 4

Ingredients:

- 2 tablespoons olive oil
- 2 garlic cloves, minced
- ½ cup veggie stock
- 4 cod fillets, boneless
- 1 cup cherry tomatoes, halved
- 2 tablespoons lime juice
- A pinch of black pepper
- 1 tablespoon chives, chopped

Directions:

1. Heat up a pan with the oil over medium-high heat, add the garlic and the fish and cook for 3 minutes on each side.
2. Add the rest of the ingredients, bring to a simmer and cook over medium heat for 10 minutes more.
3. Divide everything between plates and serve.

Nutrition info per serving: calories 169, fat 8.1, fiber 0.8, carbs 4.7, protein 20.7

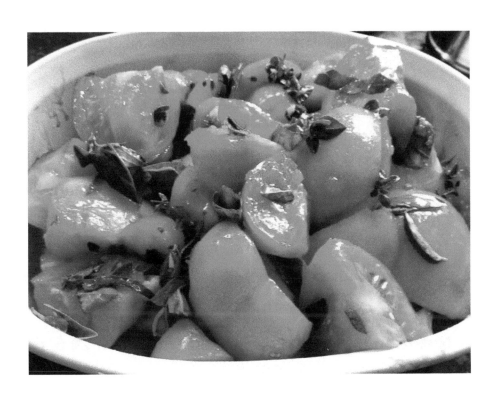

Chili Tuna

Prep time: 4 minutes ı **Cooking time:** 10 minutes I

Servings: 4

Ingredients:

- 2 tablespoons olive oil
- 4 tuna steaks, boneless
- 2 teaspoons sweet paprika
- ½ teaspoon chili powder
- A pinch of black pepper

Directions:

1. Heat up a pan with the oil over medium-high heat, add the tuna steaks, season with paprika, black pepper and chili powder, cook for 5 minutes on each side, divide between plates and serve with a side salad.

Nutrition info per serving: calories 455, fat 20.6, fiber 0.5, carbs 0.8, protein 63.8

Balsamic Cod and Spring Onions

Prep time: 5 minutes I **Cooking time:** 12 minutes I
Servings: 4

Ingredients:

- 1 tablespoon parsley, chopped
- 4 cod fillets, boneless
- 1 cup orange juice
- 2 spring onions, chopped
- 1 teaspoon orange zest, grated
- 1 tablespoon olive oil
- 1 teaspoon balsamic vinegar
- A pinch of black pepper

Directions:

1. Heat up a pan with the oil over medium heat, add the spring onions, and sauté for 2 minutes.
2. Add the fish and the other ingredients, cook for 5 minutes on each side, divide everything between plates and serve.

Nutrition info per serving: calories 152, fat 4.7, fiber 0.4, carbs 7.2, protein 20.6

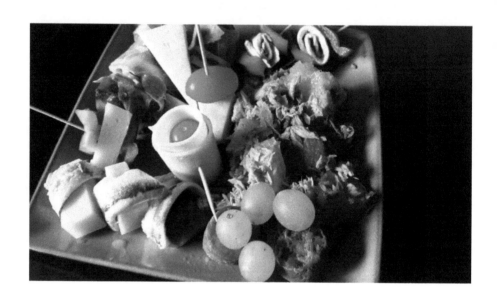